Easy Skincare Recipes for Natural Beauty

Improve Your Skincare with These Simple Recipes

Table of Contents

Introduction

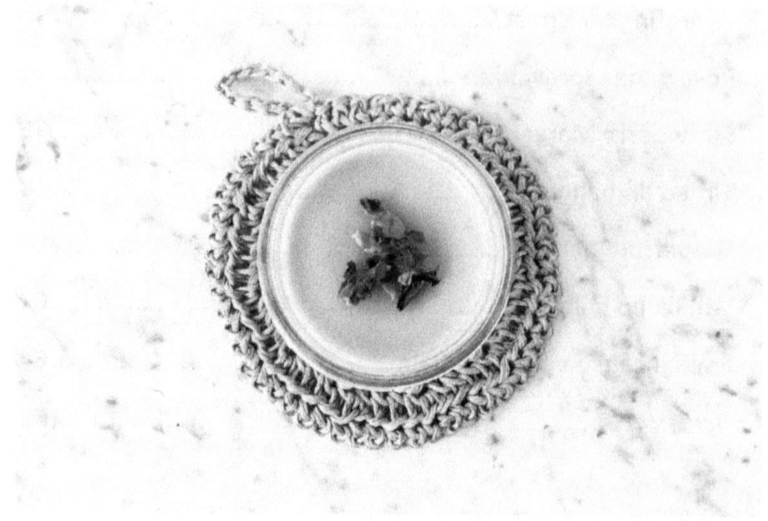

The journey to having healthy skin with even tone starts with a proper skincare routine. Most of the store-bought products promise a lot but won't do the job. The silicones present in them will clog your pores and make your skin look dull.

This is when the natural products step in to solve all of your skin problems. By using the right ones, you will manage to nourish your skin. When using natural skincare routine, the following steps are recommended:

1. Cleaning with a mild cleansing product (in the morning and evening)

2. Applying a serum

3. Hydrating your skin with a rich moisturizer.

4. Do a gentle scrub once or twice a week, to remove dead skin cells and sebum.

5. Protect your lips with a natural lip balm to avoid flakiness.

This book has every step of your natural skincare routine covered. A total of 30 recipes is here for you to choose from. You can pick the right recipe that suits your skin type.

Let's start the fun journey into natural beauty and skincare!

Rose makeup melting balm

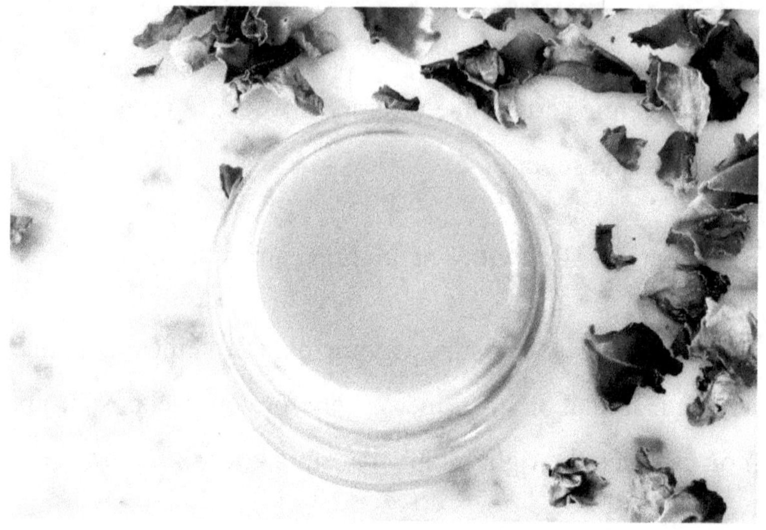

Makeup residues on your face are the number one cause for acne breakouts. That's why you need an excellent product that will melt the makeup away without drying your skin. Makeup melting balms are an excellent choice. The rich and creamy product will remove the last residues of makeup because of the presence of natural oils. Massage on dry skin using gentle circular motions. Put a hot wet washcloth over the face and gently wipe it. You can clean your skin with your usual foamy cleanser after this step.

Ingredients:

- 2 tbsp white beeswax pellets
- 1/2 cup jojoba oil
- 1 tsp Emulsifying Wax Olive Derived
- 1/8 tsp pink rose petal powder
- 1/2 tsp organic rose wax

Instructions:

1. Melt together the beeswax and emulsifying wax in a double boiler over medium heat. You can do this by filling a pot with water and place a smaller heatproof bowl that fits right over the top. Stir constantly and break the lumps.

2. When they are melted, remove from heat. Add in jojoba oil and rose powder. Mix it well and let cool for a few minutes.

3. Add the rose wax and mix until it melts. If the mixture hardens, place it over low heat. Break any lumps and mix well.

4. When it is done, pour it into a clean container. Leave it on room temperature to harden.

Lemon and honey facial cleanser

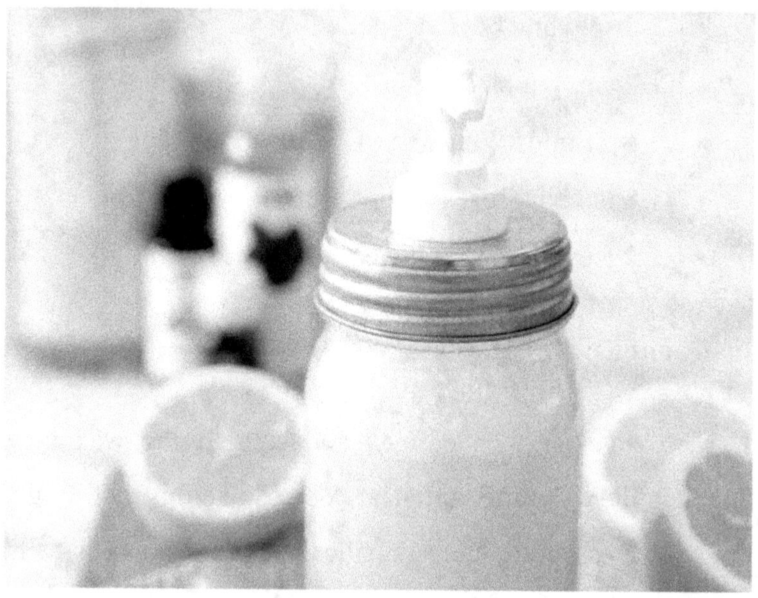

Do you want to keep the toxic ingredients away from your skin? This facial cleanser will leave your skin clean, hydrated, and free from chemicals. The glycerine is the secret ingredient that will keep your skin hydrated. You don't need to add any preservatives, as this product can last for quite a time. Whether you are an experienced cosmetic maker or a beginner, this recipe is a no-fail one.

Ingredients:

- 3 tablespoon honey
- ½ cup vegetable glycerine
- 4 drops lemon essential oil
- 2 tablespoons liquid castile soap

Instructions:

1. In a small bowl, mix the ingredients carefully.

2. Pour into a clean container of your choice. To clean your skin, apply, and massage for at least 30 seconds. Use gentle circular motions to make sure that your skin is perfectly clean. After that, rinse with lukewarm water.

Oil-based face cleansing balm

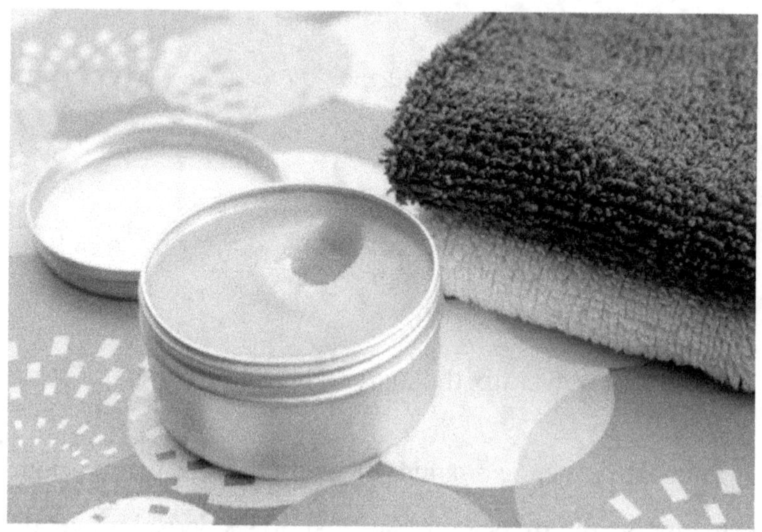

Oil might not seem like the perfect facial cleanser to you. But professionals would say that oil attracts oil. And there is no better way to clean your face than this completely natural cleansing balm. It will deep clean the pores and balance the skin's natural production of oils.

Keep in mind that this recipe can be an excellent face mask or cuticle balm too!

Ingredients:

- 1 tablespoon coconut oil
- 2 tablespoons shea butter

- 1 teaspoon calendula oil

- 1 tablespoon solid cocoa butter)

- 5 drops frankincense essential oil

- 5 drops geranium essential oil

- 5 drops bergamot essential oil

Instructions:

1. Mix the shea butter, coconut oil, and cocoa butter in a microwave-safe bowl.

2. Microwave for 30 seconds. Remove and stir.

3. Put it back in the microwave on 30 seconds. Repeat the process until all of your ingredients are well mixed and melted.

4. Let it cool for a little bit, but not completely. Add the rest of the oils and mix well.

5. Pour the cleansing balm into a clean jar. Wait for it to harden before using.

Gentle face foaming wash with jojoba oil

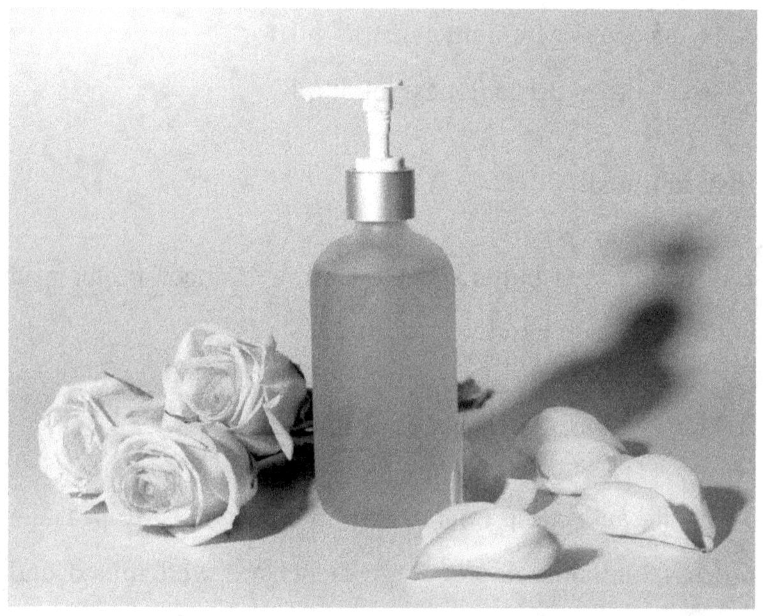

Are you looking for easy and cheap facial cleansers? This recipe will amaze you. The foamy wash with jojoba oil will clean the excess dirt and sebum from your skin and prepare it for the following steps of your skincare routine. The secret ingredients are castile soap, which will remove dirt without stripping your skin from its natural oils. You won't get the dry and flaky feeling that you normally get when using storebought products.

Ingredients:

- 2/3 cup distilled water
- ½ tsp. jojoba oil
- 1/3 cup unscented liquid castile soap

Instructions:

1. Mix together all of the ingredients. You can use boiled water if you don't have distilled water handy.

2. Take a clean foamy soap dispenser. Pour in your homemade facial cleanser. This will allow you to get the right amount you need for every wash easily. To clean your face, start with wet skin. Apply one or two pumps on your hands and gently massage your face. Rinse with warm water.

Chamomile face wash

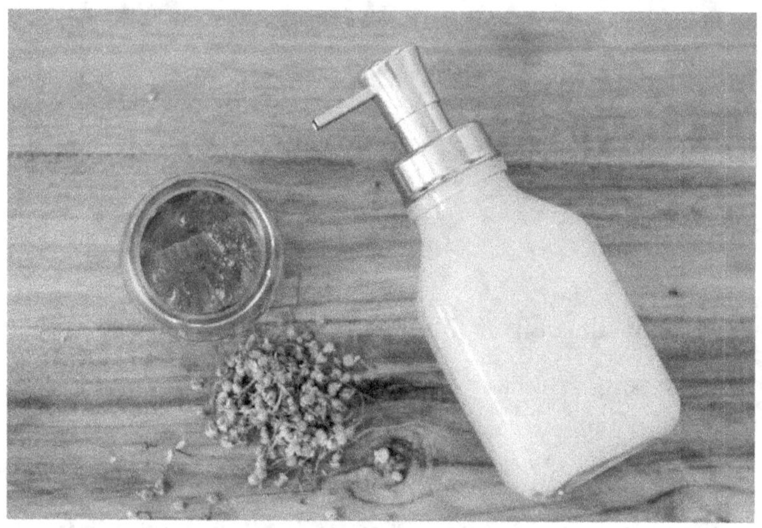

Are you looking for a rich cleanser that is suitable for sensitive skin too? Chamomile is the secret ingredient in this face wash recipe. It will help heal scars, irritations, and has antibacterial properties. Together with honey, they form the best combo ever.

Ingredients:

- 1 3/4 cup of Filtered Water
- 1/2 cup of Unscented Castile soap
- 8 tsp Almond Oil
- 2-3 tbsp Honey
- 1.5 tbsp Dried Chamomile Flowers

- 12 drops of Melaleuca Essential Oil

- 12 drops of Lavender Essential Oil

- 8 drops of Rosehip Seed Oil

Instructions:

1. Start by preparing chamomile-infused almond oil. In a double boiler, heat up the oil. Add in the dry chamomile, and heat for 30 minutes. Stir occasionally.

2. Using a cheesecloth, strain the oil.

3. In a clean glass dispenser, add the water. Add the soap after the water.

4. Pour in the infused almond oil. Screw the lid and shake until combined.

5. Add in the honey and essential oils. Shake again.

Anti-aging eye treatment with honey and rosehip

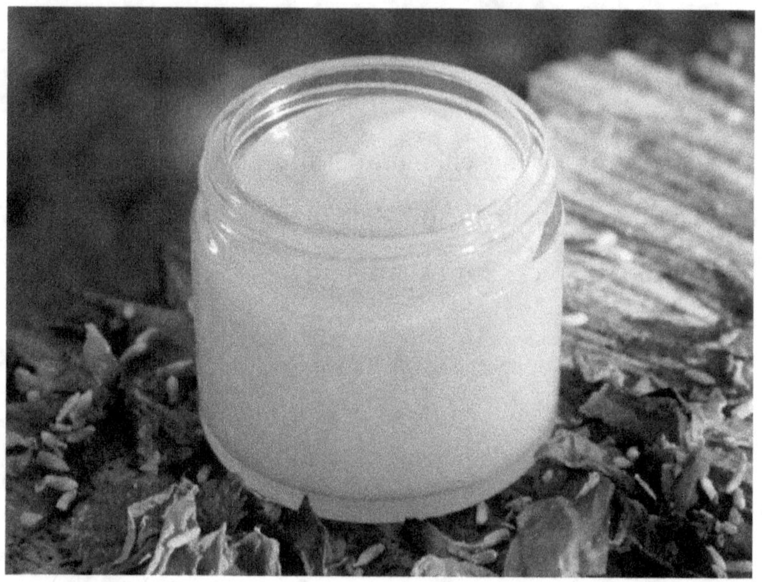

The skin around under your eyes is so thin, which means that it is more vulnerable. This eye cream has a carefully picked selection of rich ingredients. Rosehip seed oil is excellent for wrinkles and dry skin, while sweet almond oil will make the skin smooth.

Ingredients:

- 6 tablespoons sweet almond oil
- 1/2 tablespoon raw honey

- 2 tablespoons beeswax

- 3 drops of lavender essential oil

- 2 tablespoons rosehip seed oil

Instructions:

1. Add the beeswax and sweet almond oil in a heatproof bowl. Melt over a double boiler, in a heatproof bowl.

2. When the beeswax is all melted, remove the bowl from the heat and let it cool slightly. Add the honey and constantly stir for one minute.

3. Add the essential oils next. Stir well and let it cool until thickened. Then, stir again. You would want to give it a good mixing. Transfer to a clean container. Keep it in a dry place for up to three months.

Caffeine eye serum for instant wake up

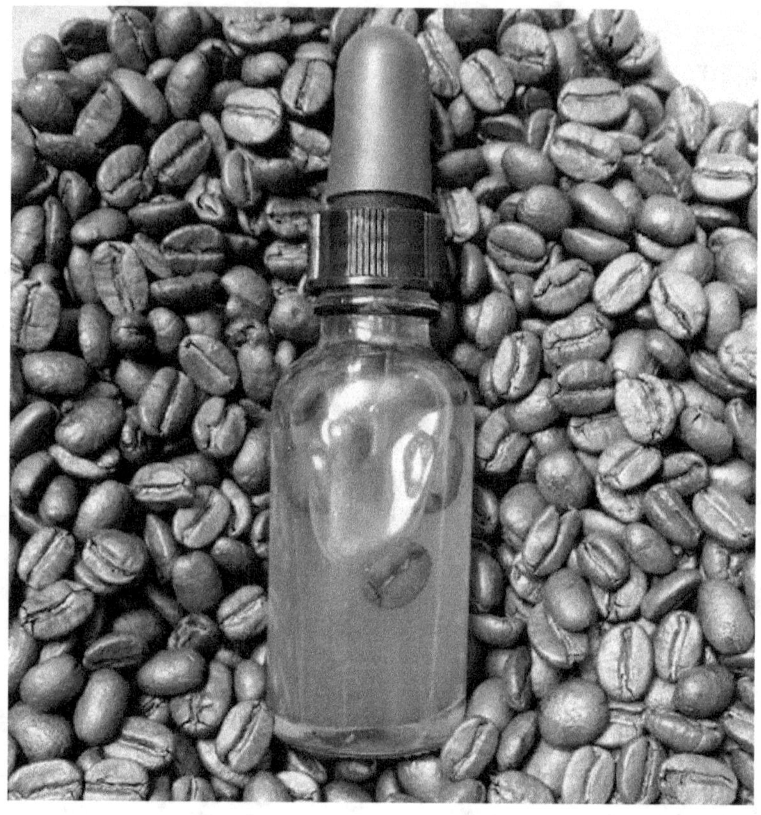

This caffeine eye serum has the power to fight puffy eyes. You can apply it to your under-eye area, in the morning and evening. The secret ingredients caffeine is known to boost the circulation and freshen up the skin. This serum is perfect if you want to look fresh and young.

Ingredients:

- 1/4 cup ground organic coffee
- 2 Tbsp castor oil
- 1/3 cup sweet almond oil

Instructions:

1. The first step is to prepare a coffee-infused oil. In a glass jar, mix the almond oil and coffee. Cover and let it sit for 1 week.

2. Strain the infused oil using a cheesecloth.

3. Add in the castor oil. Mix well.

4. Using a small funnel, pour the serum into a clean dropper bottle. Or for a better effect, pour it into a roller bottle with a metal ball. The cold metal ball will instantly reduce the puffiness.

Anti-wrinkle eye serum

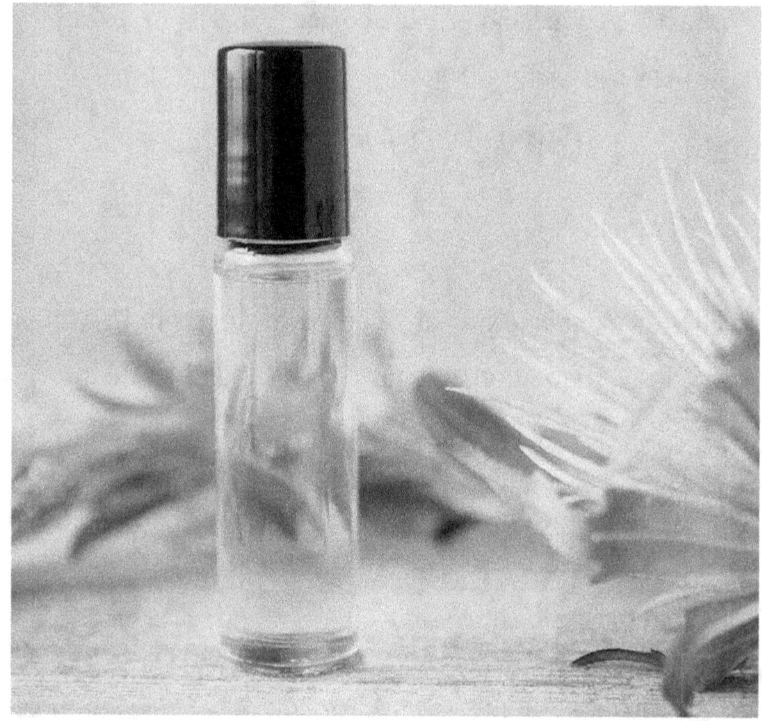

This serum recipe contains the right proportion of essential fatty acids. They will moisturize and nourish the skin, fighting the dryness and dehydration. It will reduce the fine lines, wrinkles, and dark circles. The best thing is that any skin type can use it.

Ingredients:

- 1 teaspoon Rose Hip Oil
- 1 teaspoon Evening Primrose Oil
- 3 drops Vitamin E
- 15 drops Carrot Seed Essential Oil

Instructions:

1. In a clean roller bottle, add the primrose oil.

2. Then, add in the Vitamin E and essential oil.

3. Lastly, add the rosehip oil in the bottle. Carefully, put the roller on the top. Mix the container so that the oils will combine. Apply it on the undereye area and lightly dab with your fingers. Repeat each morning and evening on clean skin.

Glowing skin serum with vitamin C

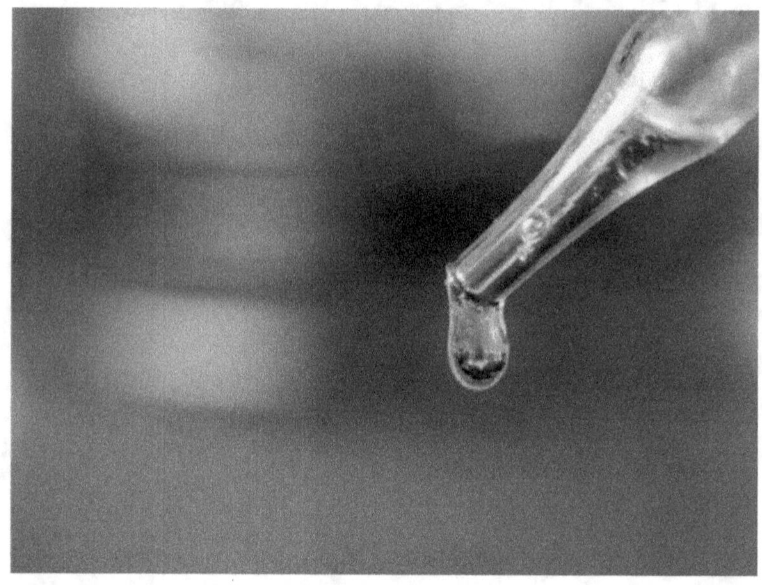

Vitamin C is the secret ingredient for high-quality homemade skin serum. It will instantly freshen up and tighten the skin. You will look younger, and your skin will have a healthy glow. When you use this serum often, you will achieve an even complexion. You won't need to put a foundation to have perfect skin.

Ingredients:

- 1 teaspoon Vitamin C Powder
- 2 Tablespoon Vegetable Glycerine
- 1 teaspoon Distilled Water

Instructions:

1. In a bowl, add the vitamin C powder.

2. Pour in the water. Mix well so that the powder vitamin C is completely dissolved.

3. Add the glycerine. Mix again so that everything is well combined.

4. Pour the mixture into a bottle dropper using a small funnel. It can last in the fridge for about two weeks, or one week at room temperature. Apply on clean and dry skin. Continue and apply your favorite moisturizer.

Moisturizing Green tea serum

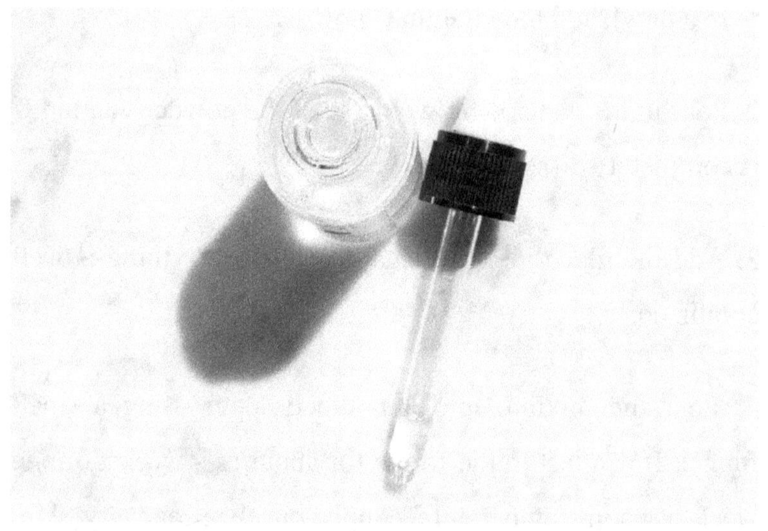

If you are looking for a good skin serum that will fight the dryness during cold months, this is your recipe. The infused olive oil will offer your skin with moisture and prevent it from getting flaky. It is suitable for mature and sensitive skin too.

Ingredients:

Infused oil:

- 1 2/3 cups extra virgin olive oil
- 1 cup of organic green tea

Serum:

- 1/4 cup avocado oil
- 1/4 cup jojoba oil
- 12 drops rosemary essential oil
- 1/8 cup sunflower oil
- 12 drops lavender essential oil
- 4 drops myrtle essential oil
- 8 drops geranium essential oil

Instructions:

1. Add the green tea in a clean and dry glass jar.

2. Cover with the olive oil. Close the lid and let the oil absorb the ingredients from the green tea. The process will take from 4 to 6 weeks. Shake the jar regularly to mix the ingredients and make sure that the tea is covered with oil.

3. Strain with cheesecloth. Pour the oil into a clean jar.

4. Add in the rest of the ingredients. Shake well to combine.

5. Pour the serum in a dark bottle to preserve it from light. Store in a cool and dark place. It will last for several months.

Face lotion for sensitive skin

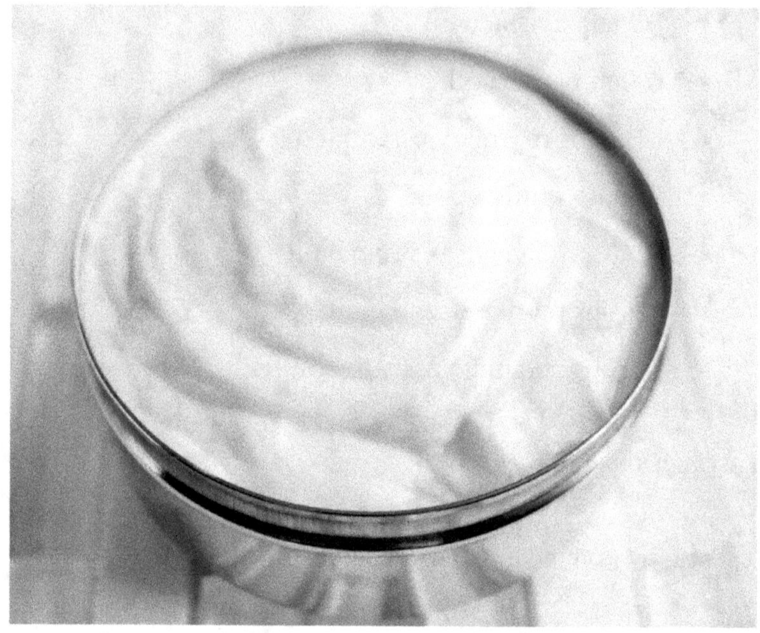

Here is a perfect recipe for lotion for your sensitive skin. This lotion contains rich oils that are perfect for soothing sensitive and dry skin. The aloe vera will reduce skin inflammations, and the apricot seed oil will nourish the skin without feeling greasy and heavy.

Ingredients:

- 3 Tbsp Apricot Kernel Oil
- 3 Tbsp Shea Butter
- 1 tsp Aloe Vera Gel

- 1 tsp Vitamin E
- 5 drops Myrrh Essential oil
- 3 drops Clary Sage Essential oil
- 5 drops Helichrysum Essential oil

Instructions:

1. Whip the shea butter using a hand mixer. When it is all fluffy, add the apricot kernel oil.

2. Add aloe vera, vitamin E, and the essential oils. Mix again until combined.

3. Store in a clean container in a dry and cool place. The lotion will last for 6 to 12 months.

Anti-aging moisturizer

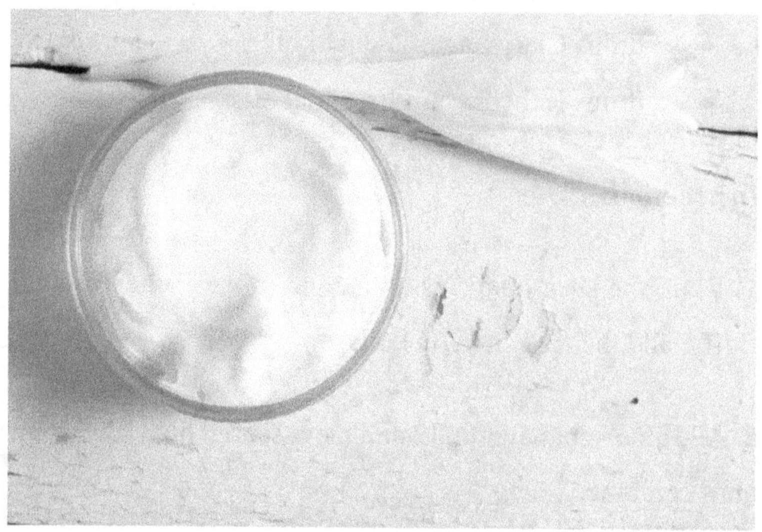

This face moisturizer will hydrate and repair your skin. The nourishing oils will improve the skin tone and texture. Avocado oil can be absorbed deeply into the skin layers and offer maximum moisturizing abilities. Pomegranate seed oil stimulates the skin to revive and fights against damage.

Ingredients:

- 2 tablespoon pomegranate seed oil
- 2 tablespoon avocado oil
- 10 drops frankincense essential oil

- ¼ 15 drops rose essential oil cup meadowfoam seed oil
- ½ teaspoon vitamin e oil
- 2 tablespoon emulsifying wax NF
- 1 cup pure rose water
- ¼ teaspoon Saliguard PCG

Instructions:

1. Melt wax together with pomegranate seed oil and avocado oil over a double boiler.

2. In a second double boiler, heat the rose water.

3. When both mixtures are the same temperature, add the rose water into the oils.

4. Mix with a hand blender for 40 seconds to 1 minute. Let it cool for 15 minutes. Then, mix for 30 seconds or until the water no longer separates.

5. Cool down the mixture slightly. Add in essential oils and vitamin e.

6. Add in the Saliguard preservative. Mix with a spoon.

7. Pour into a container and let it thicken for 24 hours.

Soothing face moisturizer for mature skin

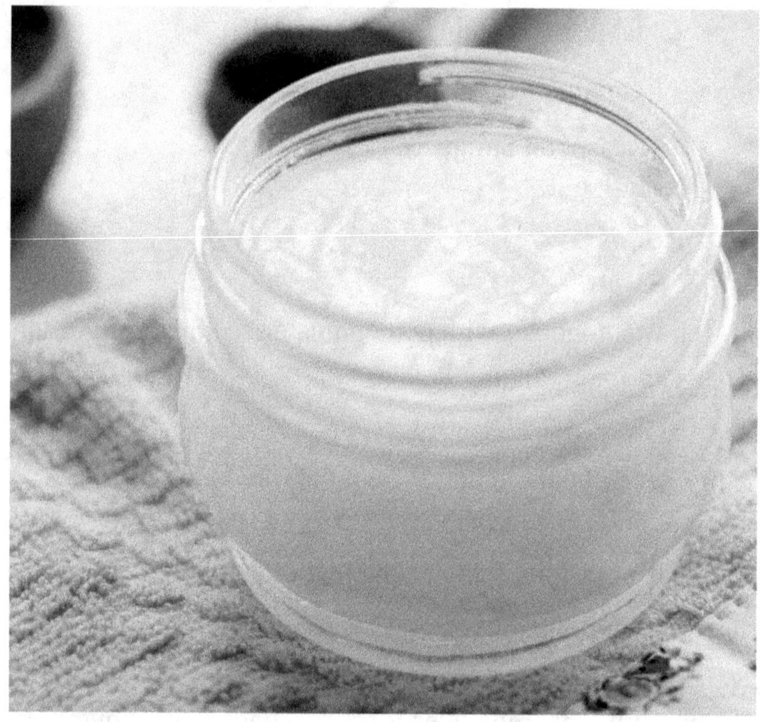

The secret ingredient in this face cream is the lemon essential oil. It is rich in vitamin C, which fights against oxidation. And we know that this is the reason for skin aging.

Ingredients:

- ¼ cup Shea Butter
- ¼ cup Coconut Oil

- 1 tablespoon Argan oil

- 1 teaspoon Vitamin E

- 10 drops of lavender essential oil

- 5 drops of lemon essential oil

Instructions:

1. Take two microwave-safe dishes. Pour coconut oil in one, and shea butter in the seconds. Put in the micro until melted.

2. In a bowl, combine the separately melted oils with argan oil and vitamin E. Mix well.

3. Add the essential oils and mix again. Pour into a clean container and let it cool completely.

Non-greasy aloe vera face moisturizer

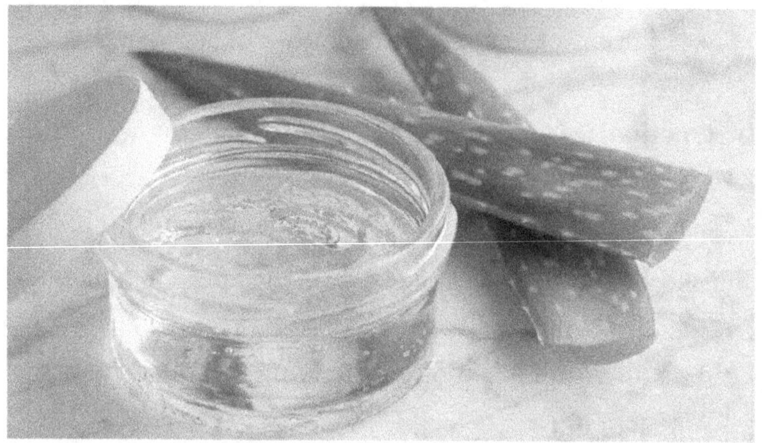

Thinking that the oily skin doesn't need a moisturizer is very wrong. Every skin type needs a dose of hydration. When it comes to oily skin, you will need a light moisturizer that won't grease your skin. This recipe will reveal the recipe for the perfect aloe vera face moisturizer for healthy skin.

Ingredients:

- 1 teaspoon jojoba oil
- 2 tablespoon aloe vera gel (use the cosmetic aloe vera, not fresh)
- 3 drops turmeric essential oil
- 3 drops lavender essential oil

Instructions:

1. In a large container, pour in the aloe vera gel. Keep in mind that this recipe won't work well if you use pure aloe vera instead of cosmetic aloe vera.

2. Add in the jojoba oil and mix until it gets fluffy.

3. Add essential oils. Mix well and store. Shelf life is five weeks.

Frankincense face cream

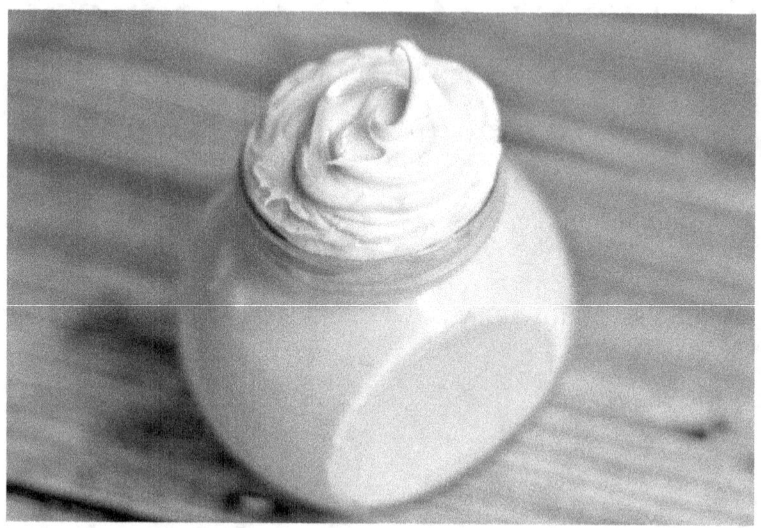

This cream is perfect for dry and sensitive skin. It will protect the vulnerable skin from any weather influence. The best thing is that you will be sure that you put 100% safe and non-toxic ingredients on your face.

Ingredients:

- 3 tablespoons jojoba oil
- ½ cup coconut oil
- 3/4 ounce beeswax pastilles
- 1 cup aloe vera gel
- 10 drops ylang ylang essential oil

- 10 drops frankincense essential oil

Instructions:

1. Melt the coconut oil, jojoba oil, and beeswax over a double boiler. Keep the temperature low, while continually stirring.

2. When completely melted, pour into a blender. Let it cool and slightly harden.

3. Then, mix with a fork. Add one tablespoon of the aloe vera gel.

4. Blend on high for half a minute. Add in some more aloe vera, blend again, and add aloe again. This way, it will combine with the rest of the mixture.

5. Blend for several minutes until thickened.

6. Add in the essential oils and blend until they are well mixed. Pour into a container and use it on clean skin.

Rich night cream

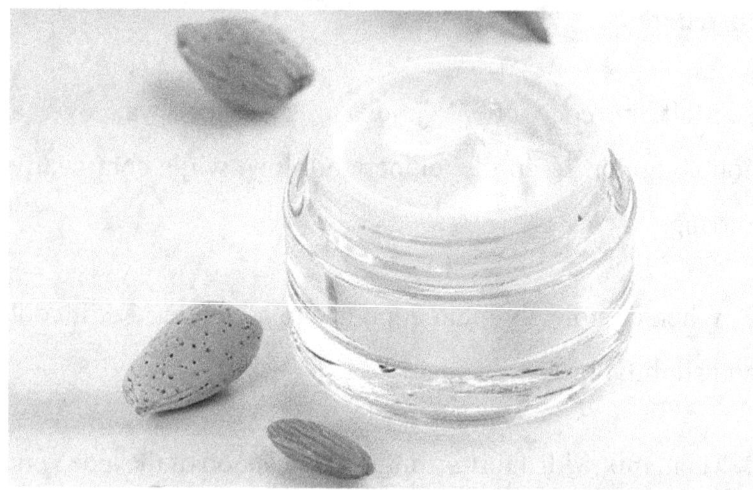

During the night, your skin will replenish itself. You need to clean it in the evening and apply a rich night cream. This cream will detoxify and brighten your skin, leaving it with a radiant and healthy glow in the morning. Apply this night cream on cleansed skin before you go to bed for fantastic results in the morning.

Ingredients:

- 1/2 tsp beeswax
- 2 tbs almond oil
- 1 tsp coconut oil
- 1/4 cup aloe vera gel

- 1/2 tsp of shea butter

- 1 tsp vitamin e oil

- 1 tsp honey

- 7 drops lemon essential oil

- 1/2 tsp bentonite clay

Instructions:

1. Melt together the beeswax, almond oil, coconut oil, and shea butter. You can choose between melting in the microwave or using the double boiler method.

2. Pour it in the blender and let it cool there.

3. In a bowl, mix together aloe vera gel, lemon essential oil, vitamin E, and honey.

4. Stir the first mixture in the blender with a fork. Add the aloe vera mixture in and blend.

5. Pour into a non-metal bowl. Add the bentonite clay and mix it with a wooden spatula.

6. Pour into a container and store it in a dry place.

Deluxe rose face cream

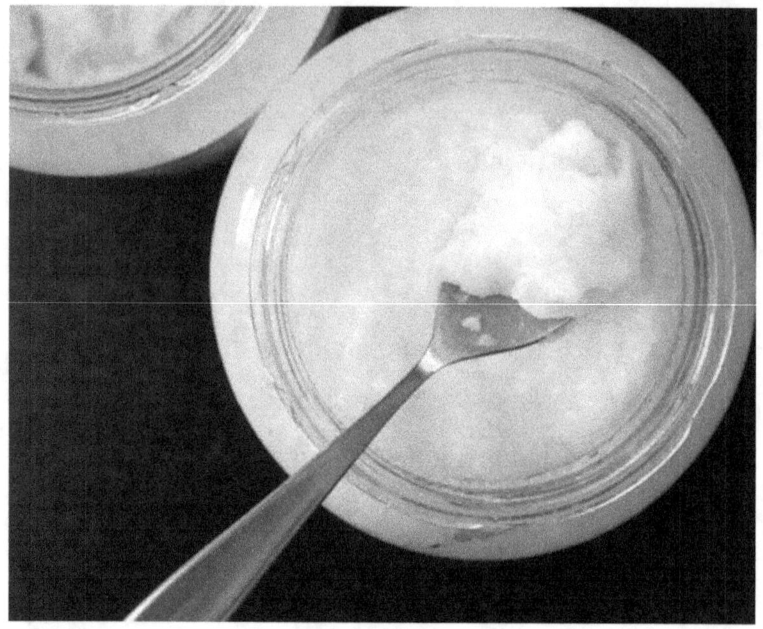

Despite their wonderful smell, roses have other benefits too. This face cream embraces all of them in favour of your skin. Rosewater is known to balance the skin's PH. It will also tone the skin and help fight acne.

Ingredients:

- 4.5 oz rose-infused oil
- 2.5 oz rose water
- 1 tablespoon beeswax
- 1/4 cup coconut oil

- 1/8 teaspoon lanolin

- 10 drops of rose essential oil

Instructions:

1. Melt together beeswax, coconut oil, and rose-infused oil over a double boiler.

2. In a second pan, heat the rose water and lanolin. When it is combined, add it slowly in the first bowl. Mix constantly.

3. Add essential oils and mix well again.

4. Store in a clean closed container. Keep your face cream in the refrigerator for up to three months.

Apple cider vinegar face toner

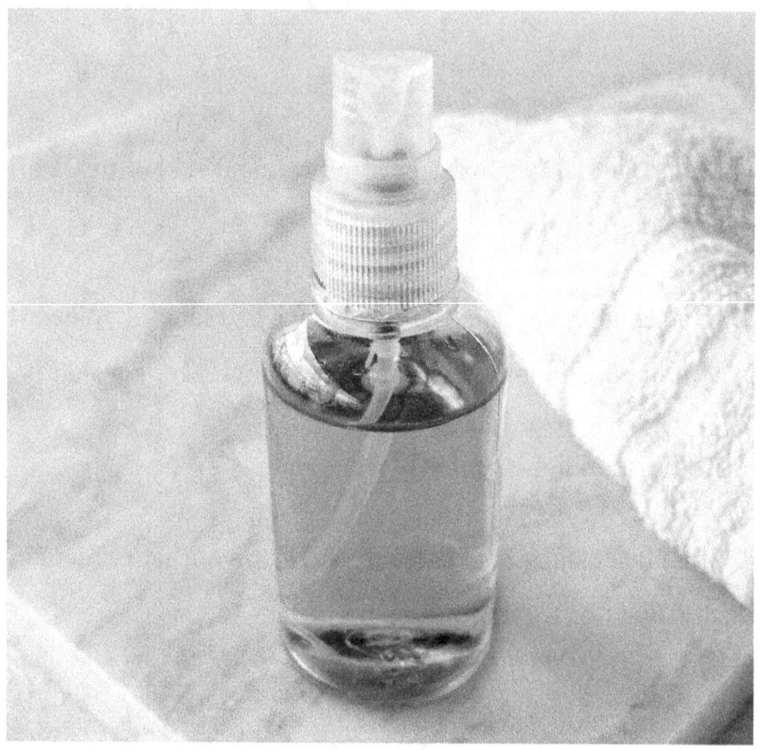

You don't need to spend your money on expensive face toners. This recipe will show you how to make one using one secret ingredient that we all have at home: apple cider vinegar. The vinegar will gently exfoliate your skin, break down excess skin oil, restore the natural pH value, and fight against acne.

Ingredients:

- 1 oz apple cider vinegar
- 3 oz distilled water
- 7 drops peppermint essential oil
- 7drops melaleuca essential oil

Instructions

1. Take a clean 4 oz spray bottle. Add all of the ingredients for the toner. Close it and shake well until combined.

2. Remember to shake the toner before each use, so that the essential oils will mix up. Close your eyes and spray on clean skin. Then, you can apply your face cream.

Natural toner for fighting acne

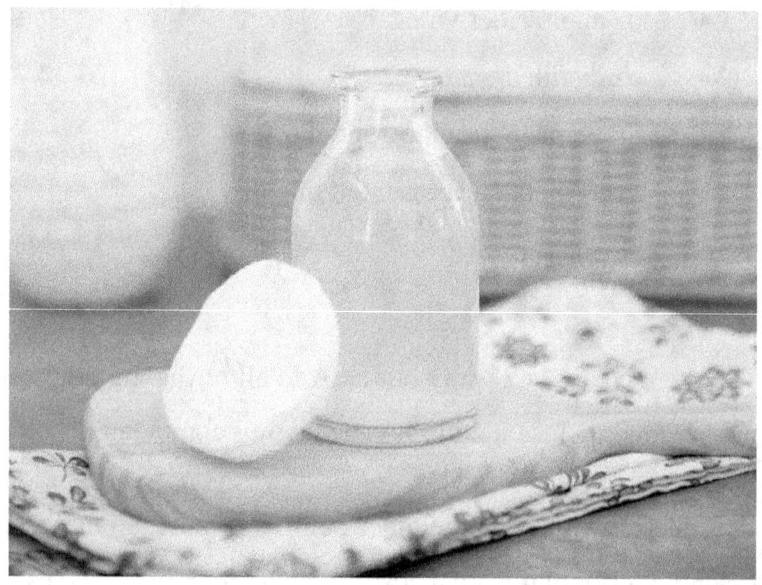

A good toner will help you disinfect your skin but in a gentle way. This will kill the bacteria on your skin and prevent acne. The number one natural skin disinfectant is vinegar. Now, you can make your own skin toner.

Ingredients:

- 2 tbsp apple cider vinegar
- 1/2 cup distilled water
- 10 drops of lemon essential oil
- 1/2 cup witch hazel

- 10 drops tea tree essential oil

- 10 drops lavender essential oil

43

Instructions

1. Pour the ingredients in a clean bottle. Shake it well.

2. Start with clean skin. Pour toner on a cotton ball and apply it to your face with gentle circular motions. It will take about 2 weeks for the results to show off.

Green tea and rose water face toner

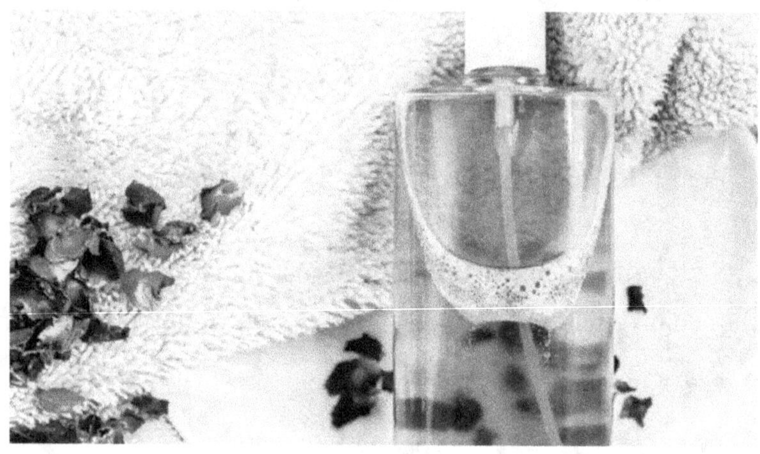

This toner gathers two of the most powerful **Ingredients:** green tea and rose water. Green tea will reduce redness and minimize the effect of the environment on your skin. Rosewater will ton the skin and give it a nice glow.

Ingredients:

- 1/4 cup witch hazel distillate
- 1/2 tsp organic green tea
- 1/2 tsp organic vegetable glycerine
- 1/2 cup rose water

Instructions:

1. In a clean jar, mix the witch hazel and green tea. Close and shake well. Leave it to infuse for two weeks. Shake daily. Once finished, stray it.

2. Pour the infused witch hazel into a bottle. Add in the remaining ingredients. Shake well.

3. Apply on clean skin, then follow with serum and moisturizer.

Natural toner for glowing skin

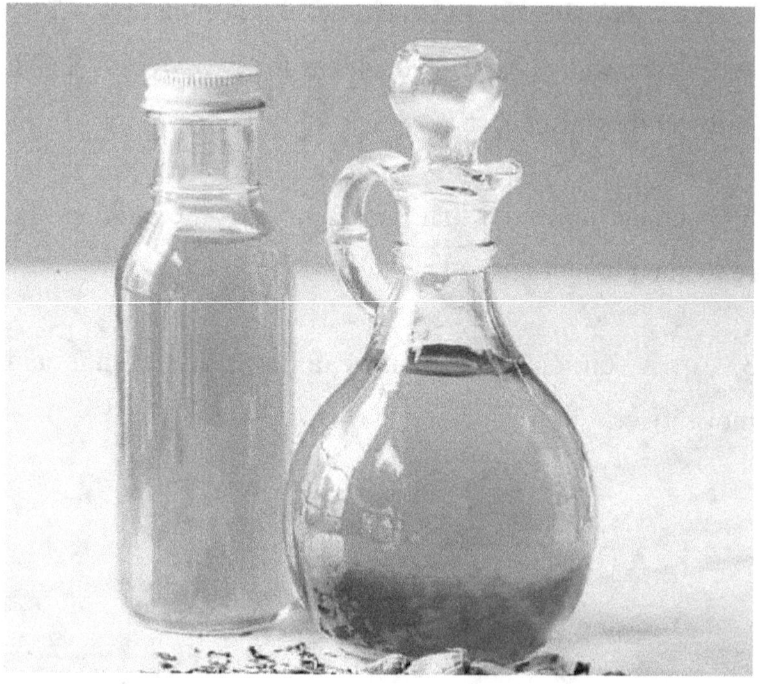

Having glowing skin has become a huge trend. However, keep in mind that it requires a good skincare routine to achieve that. When your skin is clean, nourished, and well cared for, it will give the best results. This natural toner will add the healthy radiant glow to your skin.

Ingredients:

- 1 tsp of Raw Apple Cider Vinegar
- 1.5 oz of Non-Alcoholic Witch Hazel

- 12 Drops Frankincense Essential Oil

- 12 Drops Lavender Essential Oil

- 12 Drops Lemongrass Essential Oil

Instructions

1. In a clean bottle, pour in the vinegar and witch hazel.

2. Add in the essential oils. Close the lid. Shake well so that the oils are mixed into the toner.

3. Apply with a cotton ball on clean skin. Follow up with your usual face serum and moisturizer for a full glow.

Honey and oatmeal face scrub and mask

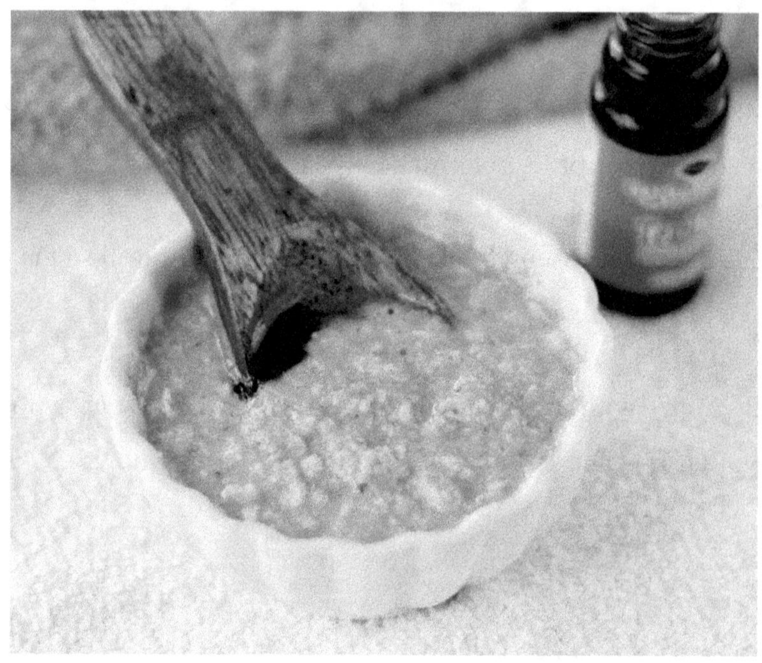

A gentle scrub will remove away the dead cells. This will leave your skin glowy and your pores clean. But, you should do only gentle scrubs on your face. This recipe is perfect and will save you some money on store-bought products.

Ingredients:

- 3 tablespoon honey
- 2 tablespoon rolled oats

- 2 drops of Peppermint Essential Oil

- 10 drops of pomegranate seed oil

Instructions:

1. Ground the oatmeal in a food processor.

2. In a bowl, mix all of the listed ingredients.

3. Start with clean skin. Apply the scrub with gentle circular motions. Massage your face with the fingertips for 2 to 3 minutes. Then, leave it as a mask for 30 minutes. It is recommended that you repeat 2 to 3 times a week for the best results.

Hibiscus and blood orange face mist

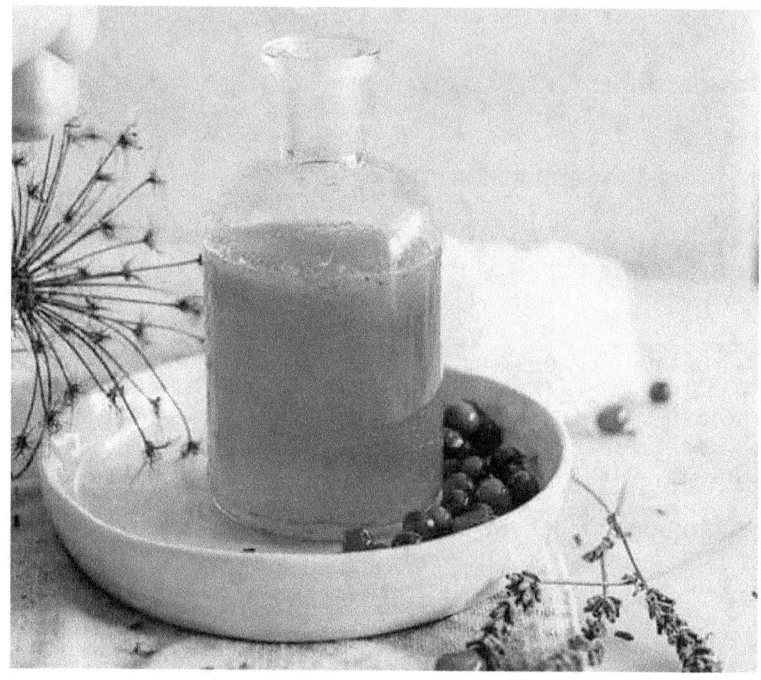

Your skin will love this mist for sure. Hibiscus will brighten your skin and even out your tone. The carefully picked mix of ingredients will boost the blood circulation and make your skin look healthy.

Ingredients:

- 2 tbsp. Blood Orange Hydrosol
- 2 tbsp. Lemon Witch Hazel
- 4 drops Lavender Essential Oil

- 2 drops Geranium Essential Oil

- 1 tsp hibiscus powder

Instructions:

1. In a clean bowl, mix the hydrosol and witch hazel.

2. Take an empty tea bag and fill it with the hibiscus. Close it and place it on top of the cup, so that it is halfway submerged.

3. Leave it for a minute. The liquid will get a nice pink color. Then remove.

4. Transfer the mist into a clean spray bottle. Add essential oils, close, and shake well.

Hydrating face mist

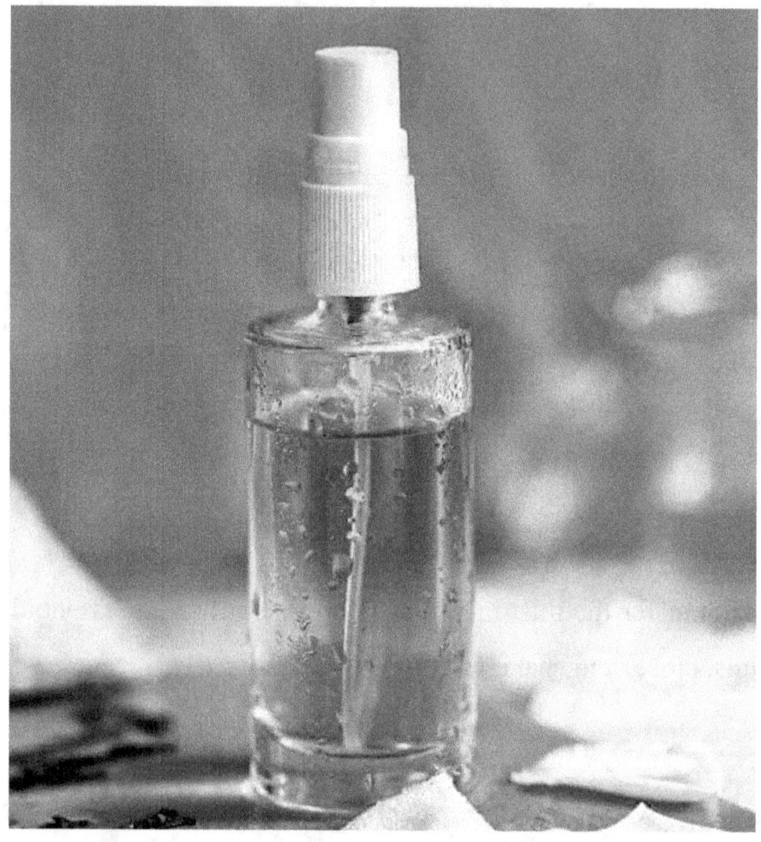

There are some moments when your skin needs excess hydration. For example, when you travel or sit under the sun for long. You can put this homemade mist in your bag and take it with you. Whenever you feel your skin is getting flakey and dry, you can spritz some on your face.

Ingredients

- 1 mint tea bag
- 8 oz water
- 1 teaspoon sweet almond oil
- 2 drop geranium essential oil
- 4 drops lavender essential oil
- 1 drop frankincense essential oil

Instructions

1. Bring the water to boil. Prepare the mint tea as directed on the package.

2. Pour the tea into a glass spray bottle, leaving space for the oils.

3. Add the almond oil. Then, add in the essential oils. Close and shake well. You can use this mist within a week.

Rose water spray

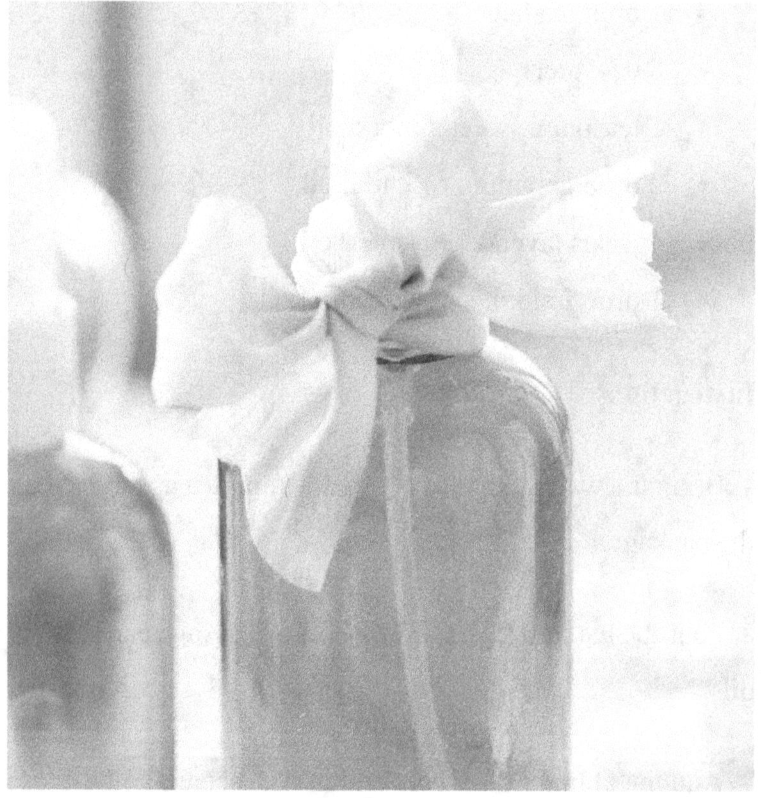

Rosewater is known to reduce inflammation, tighten pores, and soothe acne and sunburns. Also, it will tone the skin and improve its look. This spray is a must if you want to have a moisturized and healthy-looking skin.

Ingredients:

- Rose petals from 3-4 roses
- Distilled water

Instructions

1. Remove the rose petals and carefully wash them.

2. Put them into a saucepan. Cover with filtered water. Bring to simmer over medium-low heat.

3. Cover and let the petals simmer for half an hour.

4. Strain the water and throw the petals. Let the rose water cool and pour it into a spray bottle.

Strawberry Margarita lip scrub

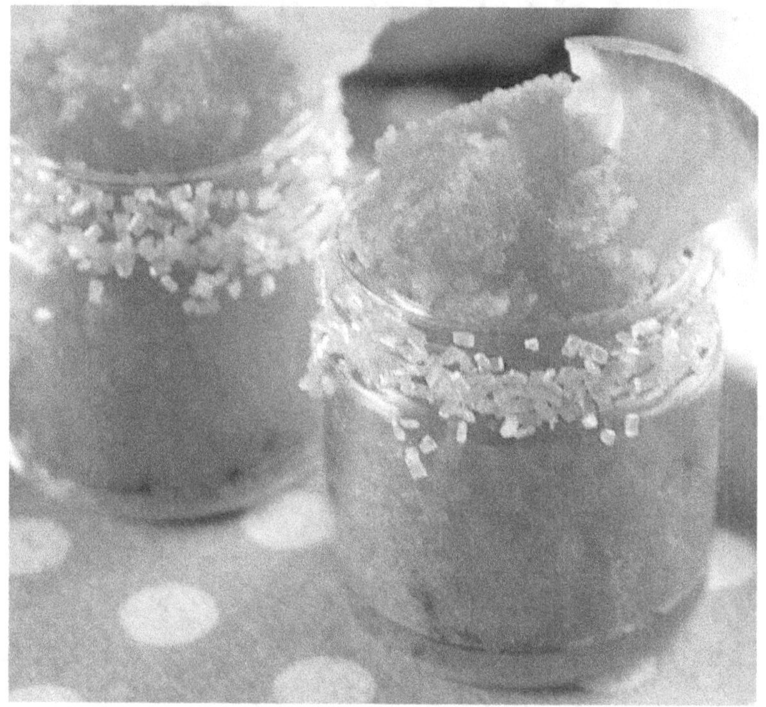

The skin on your lips is very vulnerable. Chapped lips can really look awful, so that's why you are recommended to make lip peeling. This Strawberry Margarita scrub will exfoliate your lips, leaving a nice smell. The tequila adds antiseptic properties in this recipe. This is the perfect gift for ladies too!

Ingredients

- 1/4 cup granulated white sugar
- 3 Tablespoons coconut oil
- 3-4 drops strawberry flavoring
- 1/2 Tablespoon lime zest
- 6-8 drops lime essential oil
- 2 drops Vitamin E oil
- 1/4 teaspoon tequila

Instructions

1. Add all of the ingredients for the scrub in a mixing bowl. Stir well until fully combined.

2. Transfer to clean airtight containers. Your lip scrub can last for up to three months. Apply on wet lips and massage gently. Rinse and follow up with your favorite lip balm.

Tinted lip balm

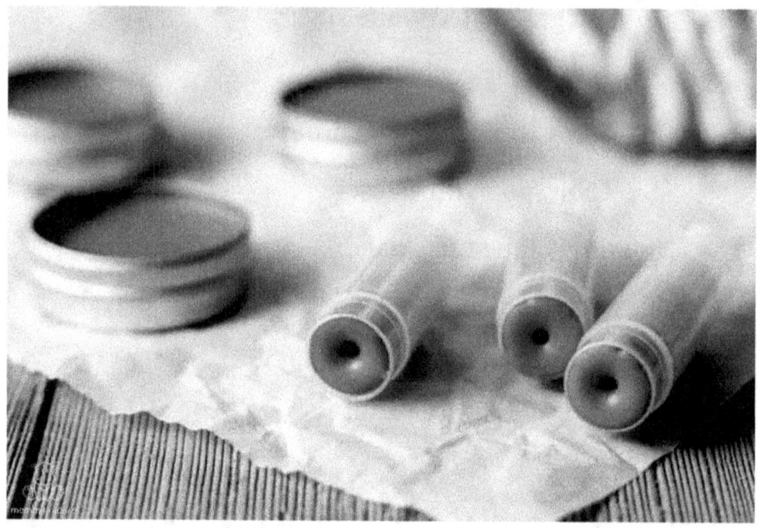

If you like to wear natural makeup, then tinted lip balm should become a part of your routine. The natural ingredients will moisturize the lips and give them a nice color. With this recipe, you can make twelve small tubes or four tins.

Ingredients:

- 1 tablespoon plus one teaspoon jojoba oil
- 2 tablespoons beeswax pastilles
- 2 tablespoons grated cocoa butter
- 1/2 teaspoon +1/4 teaspoon mica powder

Instructions:

1. Start by melting the beeswax and cocoa butter in a double boiler.

2. Pour in the jojoba oil and stir until melted and combined.

3. Add in the mica powder and stir again. Remove from the double boiler.

4. Let it sit aside for short and stir again. Then, divide the liquid among your tubes or pots and let it cool completely.

Grapefruit lip balm

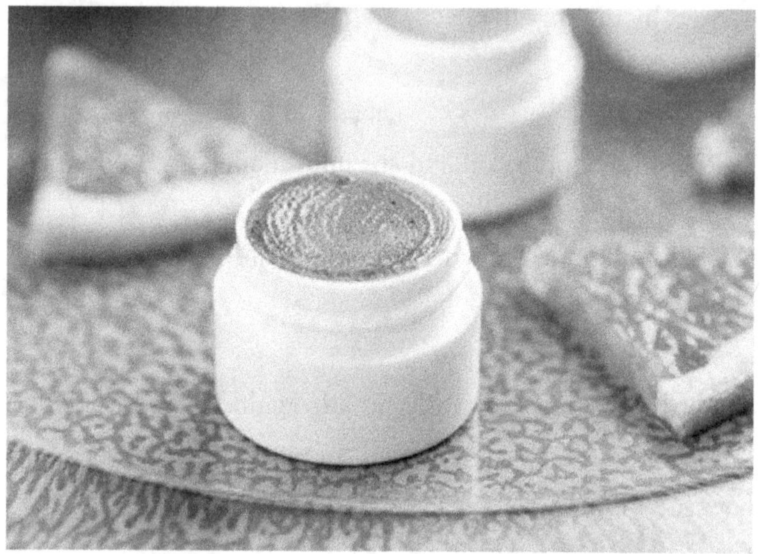

Applying lip balm is very important, and not only during colder months. The skin on the lips doesn't produce oils by itself. So, this means that you should take the care in your hands. This grapefruit lip balm smells divine and will nourish your lips as well.

Ingredients

- 1/4 cup Beeswax Pellets
- 1/4 cup Coconut Oil
- 30drops high-quality Grapefruit Essential Oil

1 tablespoon Sweet Almond Oil

Instructions

1. Before you start, have your 20 lip balm tubes ready to go. This way, you can pour them quickly.

2. Melt the beeswax together with the oils in a double boiler over low heat. Stir well.

3. Add in the essential oil. Stir well.

4. Pour into the lip balm tubes. Let them harden.

Vanilla lip balm

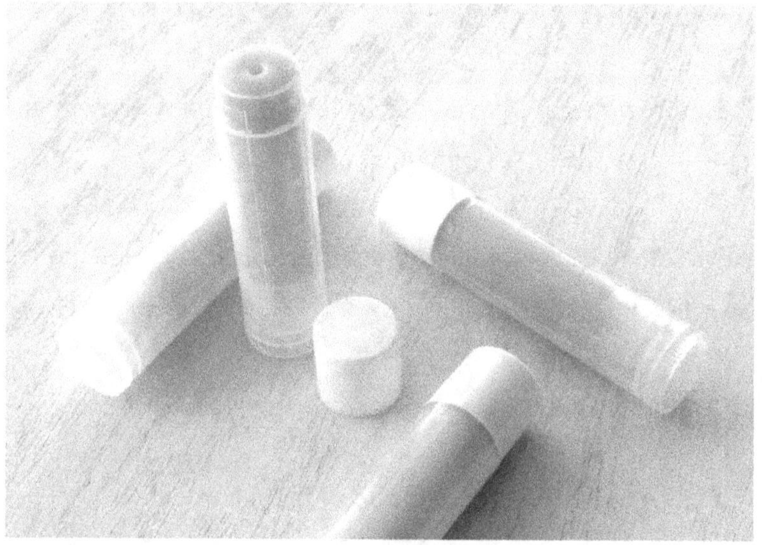

No one can resist the amazing smell of vanilla. The mix of coconut oil and shea butter will provide your lips with the needed mixture. This recipe for lip balm is very simple and easy, so feel free to prepare it even as a beginner.

Ingredients

- 2 1/4 tbsp pure shea butter
- 2 tbsp beeswax
- 2 1/2 tbsp coconut oil
- 10 drops vanilla essential oil

Instructions

1. In a microwave-safe bowl, add the beeswax, coconut oil, and shea butter. Set to medium and 1-minute interval. Remove, mix, and add for another 1-minute interval. Repeat until fully melted.

2. Then, add the essential oil. Pour the mixture into tins or tubes. Let them set for one hour at room temperature or 20 minutes in the fridge.

Frankincense Vegan Lip Balm

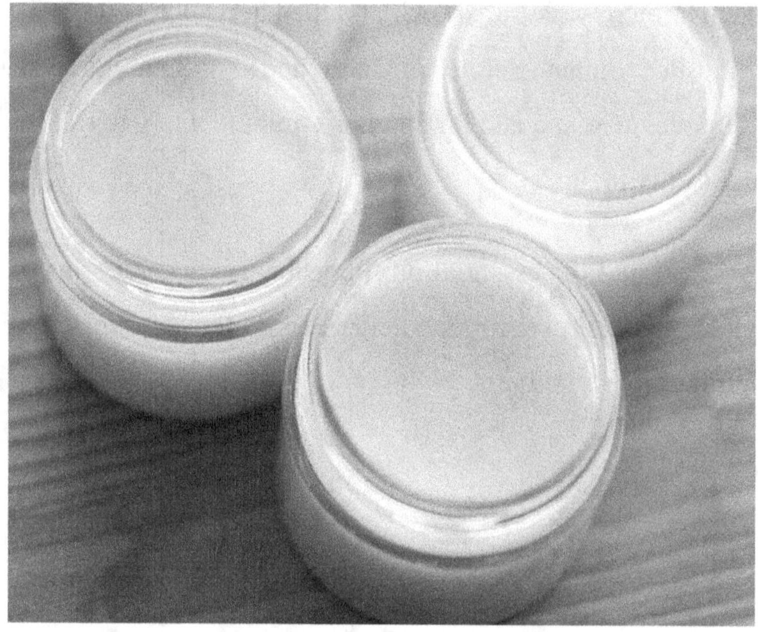

The combination of frankincense and lavender essential oils will create a divine smell. Don't forget to apply a generous amount of this lip balm before you go to bed. You will wake up to smooth and plump lips in the morning.

Ingredients

- 1 Tbsp Calendula-infused Safflower
- 3/4 Tbsp Candelilla Wax
- 3 drops Lavender Essential Oil
- 1/2 Tbsp Mango Butter

- 1 drop Copaiba Essential Oil

- 2 drops Frankincense Essential Oil

Instructions

1. In a double boiler, melt Candelilla wax, Calendula Oil, and Mango Butter. Stir occasionally.

2. Remove from heat and add in essential oils. Stir well.

3. Once the oils and wax are combined, pour the mixture into tins or tubes. Let your lip balms cool and harden.

Conclusion

With having these natural skincare recipes in your hands, you will get the skin that you always wanted. As you saw, each of the recipes has only natural ingredients. Our skin is the largest organ, so we must be careful with what we apply. With these skincare products, you won't have to worry about anything. Despite controlling the ingredients that you put on your skin, you will save money too. Natural beauty products can be so expensive, so why spend money when you can DIY it.

Enjoy the world of natural beauty!